HOMEMADE MEDICAL FACE MASK PATTERN

Table of Contents

HOMEMADE MEDICAL FACE MASK PATTERN 1

INTRODUCTION 4

CHAPTER 1:WHAT IS A FACE MASK? 5

CHAPTER 2. WHEN TO USE A MASK? 9

Preventing Infection Acquisition: 10

CHAPTER 3: HOW TO WEAR A FACE MASK PROPERLY: 13

How to wear a DIY face mask: 16

Filtering respiratory system 20

CHAPTER 4: HOW TO PROPERLY REMOVE YOUR MASK? 22

Uses of a medical face cover 24

CHAPTER 5: ARE MASKS EVEN EFFECTIVE? 26

Are homemade masks effective for healthcare workers? 34

CHAPTER 6: BUILDING AN EFFECTIVE FACE MASK 39

Three ways to upgrade the mask 40

What to do when you don't have sewing materials: 42

Is there the best material for a reusable face mask? 44

CHAPTER 7: WILL HOSPITALS ACCEPT HOMEMADE MASKS? 46

CHAPTER 8: GUIDELINES FOR WEARING A FACE-COVERING 50

Putting on your face covering 51

Making your cloth face mask 51

What you'll need 52

Do I need a filter? 53

Why are face masks necessary? 53

CHAPTER 9: HOW LONG DOES A DISPOSABLE MASK LAST? 54

CHAPTER 10: HOMEMADE FACE MASK 57

What is really important to know: 58

Using Homemade Face Masks Safely 59

When you choose to use a homemade face mask: 60

CHAPTER 11: TAKE THE FOLLOWING PRECAUTIONS TO PROTECT YOURSELF 61

How to properly dispose of masks in a lined garbage can: 61

CHAPTER 12: MAKING DIFFERENT FACE MASKS WITH EXPLANATIONS AND ILLUSTRATIONS 62

Origami Cotton Fabric Mask 62

Creative Cloth Mask 66

Bandana Protective Mask 68

CONCLUSION 72

INTRODUCTION

This book is all about the type of generally made mask, and use is likely to decrease viral exposure and infection risk on a population level, despite poor and imperfect adherence, personal respirators providing most protection. Masks worn by patients may not offer as high a degree of protection against aerosol transmission.

CHAPTER 1: WHAT IS A FACE MASK?

Face masks are a medical device used to prevent and reduce the risk of spreading infectious diseases. It can also be recognized as isolation, laser, dental, procedural, medical, the face masks are significant to ensure an excellent adequate and safe coverage of the nose and mouth, and have earrings or ties or bands in the back of the head. There are many models on the market, different in use, context, originality, and available in various colours. It is essential for using an FDA approved face mask.

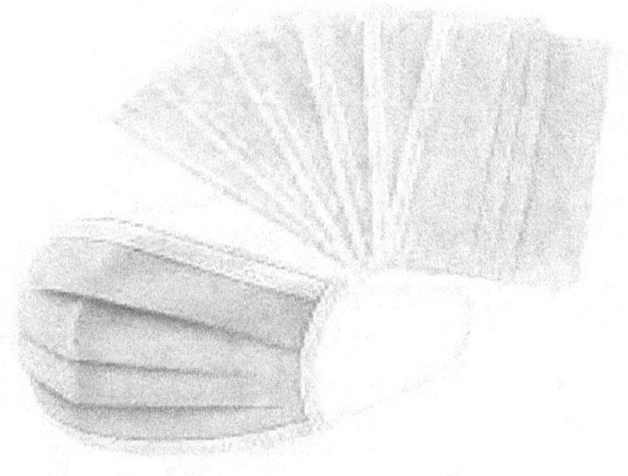

What is the use of a face mask?

Facemasks of sneezing or sprays of coughs, or other body help limit the spread of germs and bacteria. When someone talks, coughs or sneezes, they can release tiny drops of saliva into the air, that can infect others. When someone is sick, a face mask can limit the number of germs and bacteria, which would otherwise be released to the outside by breathing. So, whoever wears the cover can protect himself and other people from the risk of bacteriological contagion. Pay attention to correctly using a face mask to ensure adequate protection of the wearer' swearer's respiratory tract, so as not to come into direct contact with splashes fluids.

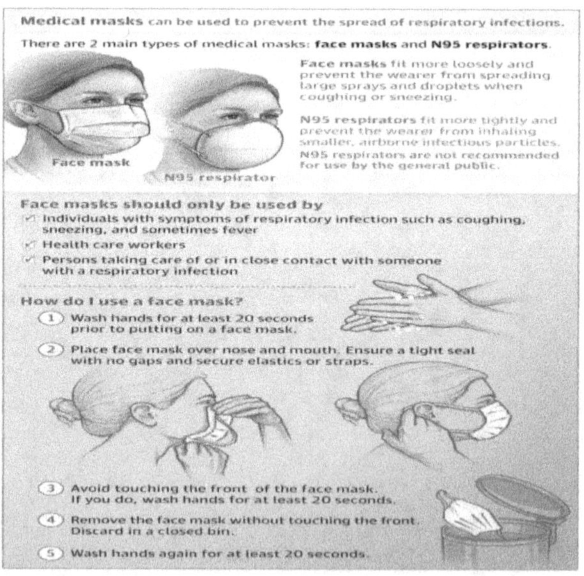

When to wear a face mask correctly?

Keep in mind that in case you are sick with cough or sneeze (with or without fever) and you know you need to get in touch together other people. Wearing the mask will help protect them from catching the disease, or spread it further in case you already have it. Healthcare settings have imposed specific rules for when people should wear face masks.

Medical masks are a Signiant medical aid, that can be used to prevent and avoid infections, which can cause respiratory problems.

This type of personal protective equipment is used to prevent the spread of respiratory infections and spread a potentially lethal virus for humanity like wildfire. These masks cover the wearer' swearer's mouth and nose and, if worn correctly, can be useful in preventing the transmission of respiratory viruses and bacteria.

There are two main models of masks considered Signiant and used against viral diseases, the prevention of respiratory infections, the so-called surgical masks, which are classed into facial and respiratory masks.

These masks differ according to the type of use for which they are intended and according to the size of infectious particles that manage to filter, and therefore not to pass. Face masks are usually suitable for viruses that cause damage to the respiratory tract. For this reason, they are particularly suitable and produced so as not to allow the transmission of these viruses, through the droplets produced by a sneeze, a cough, or even an animated discussion in tight and closed environments, where they travel short distances but are highly contagious. A classic example is the n95 respirators, which take their name from the characteristic of how they are made. They prevent access to the airways of 95% of light airborne particles. They are constructed to be perfectly adherent to the face, so as not to allow the inhalation of smaller infectious particles that can spread in the air over medium-long distances, through coughing and sneezing. There are some diseases where the use of N95 respirators is crucial. Among these diseases, the most common are tuberculosis, chickenpox, and measles. It should also be considered that for appropriate use of these particular N95 respirators must be carried out on individuals who do not have facial hair.

CHAPTER 2. WHEN TO USE A MASK?

Face masks should not be used only by people who have symptoms such as coughing, sneezing, or, in some cases, fever. Face masks should be worn primarily by healthcare professionals and by people who care for or are in close contact with patients with respiratory infections. By now we have reached the point that they must also be worn by healthy individuals to protect themselves from the acquisition of respiratory diseases because it is possible to come into contact with the so-called asymptomatic, or people who have not developed any symptoms but are healthy carriers, and a vehicle for the transmission of the virologic infection. When requests for masks intensify, to cope with emergencies, they should be reserved for those who need them most because coverages can be scarce during periods of diffuse respiratory infection. Therefore, a limited presence of masks may occur sold on the market. Because N95 respirators require specialized t testing, they are not recommended for use by the general public.

Preventing Infection Acquisition:

The perfect way to prevent the acquisition and spread of respiratory infections is to apply proper hand hygiene. Wash your hands often. Good advice suggests that you avoid touching difficult parts of disease, such as the nose, eyes, or mouth, before adequately cleaning and disinfecting your hands. Avoid close contact with other patients. Besides, appropriate cleaning of surfaces and domestic environments using special sanitizers, such as wipes or cleaning sprays.

How to wear a face mask

First of all, clean your hands with soap and water or use hand sanitizer before touching the mask.

Take off a mask from the box and make sure there are no visible tears or holes in either side of the cover.

Determine which right side of the mask is the top.

Front of the cover, which has a rigid edge bent over and intended to mould to the shape of your nose.

Determine which right side of the mask is the front.

The coloured side of the cover is usually the front and should face away from you, while the white hand touches your face.

Follow the instructions below, paying attention to the type of mask you are using.

- Face Mask with Ear-loops:
- Hold the mask by the ear loops.
- Place a circle around each ear.

Face Mask with Ties:

Carry the mask to the nose level and place the ties over the crown of the head, and secure with a bow.

Face Mask with Bands:

Hold the mask in hand with the nosepiece or top of the costume at undertips, making sure that the headbands are hung under the palms.

Carry the cover to the nose level and pull the upper strap over the head, until it sits on top of the head.

Pull the lower strap over until it rests on the nape of the neck.

Mould or pinch the hard edge to the shape of the nose. In case you are using a face mask with ties:

Then take the bottom links, one in each hand, and secure them, making a bow at the nape of the neck.

How to take off a face mask

First of all, clean your hands with soap and water or hand sanitizer before touching the mask. Avoid touching the front of the cover. The front of the hood is contaminated. Only contact the ear loops/ties/band.

How to put on a Mask

If it is required to wear a mask, it is a vital measure to sanitize the hands, mixing soap and water, and rinsing for 30 seconds, and then you can safely use it. An excellent solution sees the use of an alcohol-based disinfectant, the content of which must be at least 60% alcohol.

This method can also replace or be complementary to washing with soap and water.

After cleaning the hands, place the face mask over the nose and the mouth. Be sure to ensure an airtight seal with your face. When you are wearing the mask, do not touch it, to leave it as hygienic as possible If you do feel the face mask, wash your hands, or use hand sanitizer again. After using it, remove it without touching the front of the face mask and throw it in the trash, without letting it come into contact with objects or people. Rewash your hands after dropping the face masks.

CHAPTER 3: HOW TO WEAR A FACE MASK PROPERLY:

Likely, you've never had to worry about adequately covering your nose and mouth before you and yourself being a patient in the hospital or working in medicine or construction. With the intersection of the risk of infection, surgical face masks, as well as face cloth coverings, both those purchased online and those created at home, are acquiring greater relevance and importance in the world. They are becoming a necessity during the novel coronavirus pandemic that has affected Americans in all 50 states, and the whole world.

Experts for Disease Control and Prevention are advising everyone wears face coverings in public and leaders in communities, and single states can also be mandating that you do so.

In the last period, New York Governor Andrew Cuomo approved a new legislature asking citizens to put on a face mask when social distancing measures aren't possible, including those activities with a high risk of close contacts, such as taking a means of public transport or those essential businesses in enclosed spaces. Same shortly after that, leaders in Southern California passed similar guidelines with more donate recommendations for essential workers with increased risk of closed contact.

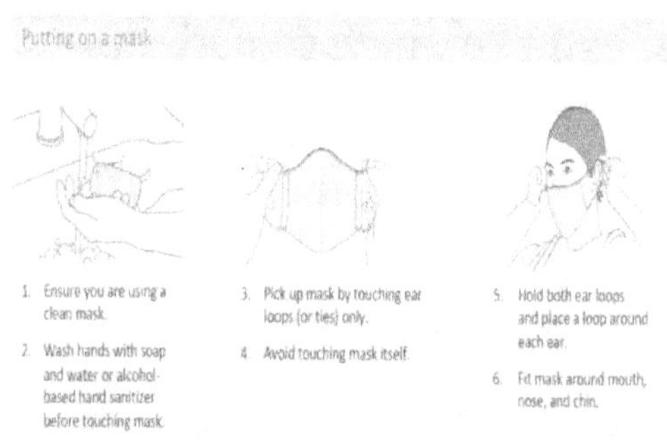

The correct way to wear a medical or homemade mask:

Bring up your mask by its ear loops. Without touching the cover, itself, bring the circuits up to your ears, securing them as tightly as possible. If the hood is equipped with ties instead of loops, tie the top pair around the lower crown of your head, and the second pair around the nape of the neck.

Be careful that it covers the nose and the mouth. The mask hinders the external emission of bacteria into the air by covering nose and mouth, wearing a medical mask correctly, it can also provide slight protection, and increase your chances of repelling any nearby particles and germs.

The mask must be adjusted so that it adheres perfectly and covers the chin, lifting it to the base of the jaw. Pulling the hood under the button is a surer way not always to have to adjust it when you leave the house, Secure the mask around the bridge of the nose. Some covers are equipped with a metal tab to be positioned at the trunk (in fact, if you feel a metal tab on the chin, you will know that the cover has been placed upside down). Make sure that the top of the mask is snug against your face. In case there is no metal tongue, make sure it doesn't slip off your nose afterwards.

While surgical masks are unable to filter all the particles and bacteria present in the air, the N95 covers are also used by healthcare professionals, so there is no need to worry about the filtering, which is guaranteed. In this case, you will only have to provide full adherence to the face to obtain effective screening.

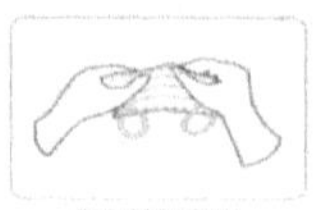
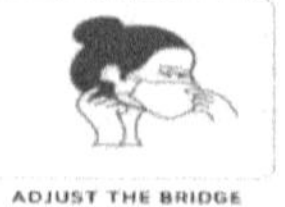
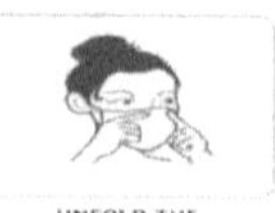

How to recognize the external side of a surgical mask?

If you have a medical-grade surgical mask, you may be wondering which side should be on the outside. Although not all manufacturers follow the same style and therefore, not all products are built in the same way, according to expert opinion, in traditional models, usually, the coloured part of the mask represents the outer side. According to Dr Rohede's view: "Looking carefully at the mask, you can consider dividing it into an "internal" and an "external" side, to understand which part should be put on the face." He also explains:

"For most surgical masks I have worn while working in public health, the colouring is turned outward."

How to wear a DIY face mask:

If you don't have a surgical mask or a hand-sewn mask, using a cloth face covering will still prevent you from spreading bacteria through droplets in public places." Dr Bearman says. "None of the masks is medical-grade, and any gaps are less important, as these are meant to prevent droplets and not aerosols. It has been widely demonstrated how COVID-19 manages to transmit through larger particles inside droplets and not through aerosols in everyday spaces, outside hospitals." Plus, a face-covering might act as a human "dog cone" in that it reminds you to avoid touching your face.

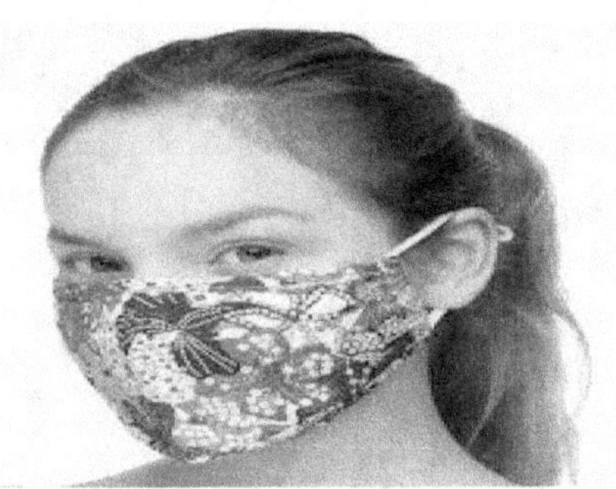

How can I clean my mask properly?

After safely removing the mask or linings by handling its ties or loops with care, Dr Bearman says that any surgical masks should be disposed of, as these are for single use only. Experts say it is wrong to attempt to disinfect surgical masks at home, although some health professionals may do it due to a shortage of supplies, all experts do not recommend doing it at home. There isn't any actual data on how you should washcloth coverings. Still, Carolyn Forte, Director of the Good Housekeeping Institute Cleaning Lab, suggests washing each mask, using hot water in washing machines, and drying in a dryer at warm temperatures.

When you intend to keep the fabric covering at home, before washing it, you should put it in a dry paper bag. According to Dr Bearman's claims, it should be ensured that any moisture contained in the masks must dry out, and therefore may not dry out properly if placed in a closed box. Dr Rohde adds that it's best to have two or three cloth masks that you can cycle between to avoid having to wash your cloth mask every time you head outside.

When and how to wear medical masks

When you take care of someone with the virus, you must take the necessary safety measures and wear a mask.

Wear a mask when you are coughing or sneezing.

Masks are a useful prevention tool, only if combined with frequent hand cleaning, rubbing it with alcohol or soap and water.

When you wear a mask, you also need to know the method on how to use it and dispose of it properly.

What to know about mask protection?

A protective mask is a device intended to protect the user from inhalation of harmful dust, pathogens, fumes, vapours, or gases. The covers and application in different sectors of use, from the military ones, from the private sector, and the public, they range from the cheapest, single-use, reusable disposable masks to replaceable cartridge models.

There are two categories of breathing apparatus, namely "filtering" device, which can be either passive or active and which force contaminated air to pass through a filtering element, and "insulating" apparatus, in which fresh air is delivered from a reserve. Within each category, different techniques are used to reduce or eliminate the harmful airborne matter. History of the development of protective Masks intended to protect against the inhalation of particles have probably been around for a long time for mining or dust sources. During epidemics of plagues, the doctors being made masks in the beak of birds called with medicinal plants supposed to kill the miasmas responsible for the contagion; In the middle of the xix the century, medical masks appear.

During the XX century, during the origins of the tanks, their occupants (pilot, gunner) were forced to wear a mask to protect themselves from the fragments of paint and metal ejected from the walls by the impacts of projectiles to the outside.

Metal protective helmets/masks with a window for vision are currently only used in metallurgy and for welding and tend to be replaced by masks made of lighter composite materials. For uses without a heat source, the plexiglass in thick sheet (1 to 5 mm) is transparent and impact resistant. Sometimes, a genuine visor made of a flexible and transparent plastic protects the face of the operator from splashes of corrosive liquid or at toxic, biological or medical risks (splashes of droplets, blood, etc.

Filtering respiratory system

Wool filter masks were used by early inventors such as Haslett and Tyndall. Wool is still used as a filter today. Wool filter masks were used by first inventors such as Haslett and Tyndall. Today wool is still used as a filter, together with other substances such as glass, cellulose, plastic, and combinations of two or more of these materials. Since filters cannot be cleaned and reused and therefore have a limited lifespan, costs and availability are key factors. There are disposable and cartridge models. Since filters cannot be cleaned and reused and therefore have a limited lifespan, price and availability are key factors. There are disposable models, as well as cartridge models.

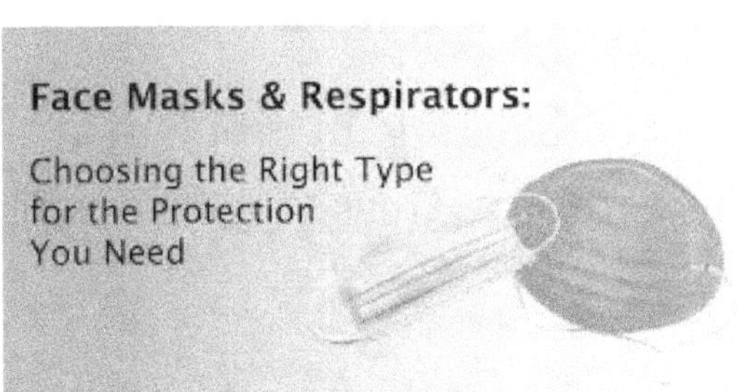

How to put on a general public mask and wear it?

First, let's remember a few instructions: the little ones should not wear a mask.

For children under 3, wearing a mask is therefore prohibited due to the risk of suffocation. The second important point, the cover is not a spacesuit; it does not protect itself from the virus and should not be seen as a free passport.

Its port must be accompanied by respect and the practice of barrier gestures.

For a mask, whether surgical or fabric, to be effective, you still have to put it on!

Several steps are to be followed carefully.

Wash the hands before putting on your mask to avoid risking soiling immediately.

Always grab it by the elastic bands to position it.

Place it well by checking in front of a mirror that covers all the essential areas: nose, mouth, but also chin.

Upon express request of the organizing committee for the Paris 2024 Olympic Games, several champions carried out video demonstrations. Here is one featuring via-time Olympic biathlon champion Martin Fourcade.

CHAPTER 4: HOW TO PROPERLY REMOVE YOUR MASK?

The steps to follow

- ➢ small freezer bag, etc.;) Have you finished your outing, or need to replace your mask for another after 4hours? Removing your cover must also obey specifics rules.
- ➢ Handle the mask only with rubber bands and remember that the outside of the cover can be potentially soiled and infected.

- ➤ Place it in an airtight box if possible while waiting for a wash.
- ➤ Wash your hands immediately.
- ➤ When it is a disposable mask, throw it away immediately, preferably in a closed bin, and, if possible, in an airtight bag in which you enclose your cover.

Washing your mask: tips and mistakes to avoid

Once your mask has been removed, it should still be washed before each new use. To clean your cover, you must comply with strict health regulations. First of all, remember that it is imperative to wash it after each use, has provided recommendations plug.

The washing of the general public fabric mask must be done in the washing machine via a cycle of a minimum of 30 minutes at 60 degrees. A scientifically validated process kills all bacteria.

First, remember to clean your washing machine, especially with bleach, to keep your drum clean. You can also spin it vacuum once at 60 degrees to kill any bacteria.

Place your masks in the drum, best to wash them separately from the rest of your laundry. You can, however, place them with old sheets if you have to clean them. If you want to spin linen with 60 degrees, you can put your masks in a dedicated bag (for example, those for lingerie).

Once the laundry is done, take out your masks and put them to dry. They must be dry after two hours of drying. If this is not the case and if you do not have a dryer, you can speed up the drying with a hairdryer.

To end out everything and avoid making mistakes regarding the maintenance of your general public mask, you can end what you are looking for in our dedicated le.

Uses of a medical face cover

The environmental protection by contaminated droplets from the potentially infected wearer, particularly in medicine and caretaking.

Protection of wearer from splashes of infectious bodily fluids, e.g., during surgery. (With appropriate additional application) Restricted protection of wearer from smear infection from unclean hands touching the mouth and nose.

What protection does the mask offer?

Most experts estimate that wearing mouth-nose protection reduces the risk of infection for other people because it captures to a specie extent droplet during talking, sneezing, or coughing. However, natural masks are not able on their own to perform efficient protection if the wearer s infected with the coronavirus. But there are also side effects. Wearing masks could ensure that people kept more distance from each other.

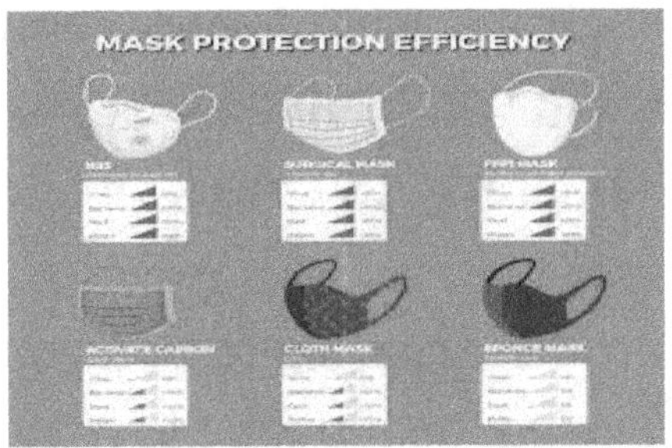

In what situations is it advisable to wear a mask?

Its recommended to wear everyday masks in public life - especially when shopping as well as on the bus and train. If a safety distance of at least 1.5 meters can be maintained or if there is alternative protection, for example, at the supermarket checkout - for instance, in partitions - then it is not necessary to wear masks.

How do I wear it?

- Masks are only useful if you wear them correctly. The WHO (World Health

Organization) has provided some essential instructions:

- Wash the hands at least for 20 seconds, using water mixed with soap before touching or wearing the mask.
- Ensure that your nose and mouth are completely covered when you wear it.
- Do not touch the mask while you are out, this in order not to contaminate it.
- Do not take off the mask while 'you're in public.
- To remove the mask once you return, untie it from the back. Don't touch the front of it.
- First of all, after returning home, you immediately wash the mask, so it doesn't contaminate your things.
- Wash your hands continuously, both immediately before putting it on and after removing it, and repeat the procedure even when you are wearing a new mask.
-

CHAPTER 5: ARE MASKS EVEN EFFECTIVE?

Some studies on homemade masks have shown that they are less effective than surgical masks and certainly cannot replace or compete for efficacy, with the first N95 respirators that health workers, who were wearing them, allow them to treat patients and take lesser risks.

Dr Koushik an internal physician, residing at the Johns Hopkins Bayview Medical Center in Maryland, says: "Homemade masks are partially effective."

They also make it possible to get a physical barrier and defend against infective particles, he said, they don't have a sound alteration system and filters as effective as those used by N95 respirators.

But compared to nothing, it is always better to have them, especially useful for those who leave the house to make a quick trip to the grocery or pharmacy, said Anna Davies and Raina MacIntyre, skilled public health researchers and authors of two separate studies on the effectiveness of cloth masks.

We need to keep in mind that masks are not able to replace the measures of social estrangement that must always exist. First, you need to keep at least six feet apart and stay home as much as possible, as this is still the best way to prevent the virus from spreading.

How do you clean them?

First, you should wash the masks both before and after each use to remove traces of any germs that you may have collected along the way. A washing method is to add the covers in a mesh washing bag and put them to wash in a washing machine so that they do not take off during washing at high temperatures, or decide to remove them directly by hand.

What if I can't make my own?

Crafters on Etsy aren't sold out with masks yet. It is difficult to understand how effective these masks are since you didn't create them yourself, but you can easily compare them with our tutorial on costumes to get an idea of what you want and then buy it: does it cover the nose and mouth? Are there folds?

Will it seal tightly around your face?

It is not necessary to purchase too many masks, given that doctors and prevention experts recommend that only one person per family be assigned to do chores and errands outside the home.

Remember that given the situation, the shipment of masks may take longer than usual, so be careful when purchasing.

Make sure you always wash your masks before putting them on.

In case you can get the masks, keep washing your hands, maintaining measures of social distancing.

Remember, staying at home is the best defence against coronavirus.

It should also be noted and taken into consideration:

Although the situation has worsened in many countries, that of putting on a face cover is advice but not an obligation.

The homemade masks do not, in any way, replace the practices of social estrangement to be adopted together with permanence in one'sone's own homes.

Despite everything, if you need to make a mask, here are some simple detailed instruction, provided by the Centers for the control and prevention of diseases, on the methods to create various models of covers, whether you know how to sew or not.

Necessary materials you'll need to make:

- Bandana, T-shirt or square cotton cloth, about 20" x 20."
- Coffee filter
- Rubber bands or hair ties

How to Make your mask

- For the screen of the mask, you'll need to cut the bottom of a folded coffee filter and keep the top.
- Start to lay a bandana or 20" x 20" T-shirt in a rectangle. Then, fold the bandana or shirt in half lengthwise.
- Then, fold the cut filter in the centre of the folded bandana or shirt.
- Now, fold the top of the bandana or shirt down over the screen. Fold the bottom up.
- In this way, place rubber bands or hair ties around the folded bandana or shirt, about 6 inches apart.
- Then fold the side of the bandana or shirt in toward the middle and tuck.
- Finally, place the rubber bands or hair ties around your ears, and voila, you've made a face mask, no sewing required.

How to sew your mask?

These are the materials you will need to get started: Tightly woven cotton fabric, to prevent germs and other impurities that are found in the air from passing through. Elastics pattern (or rubber bands, string, cloth strips, hair ties), to ensure an effective sewing system on the face.

Needle and thread (or a bobby pin, a sewing machine), scissors. All necessary tools for the correct assembly of the template.

Make your mask

- Start to cut your fabric into two 10" by 6" rectangles. Place them on top of each other.
- Then, fold over the long sides -- 1/4 inch -- and hem.
- Now, fold the double layer of fabric over 1/2 inch along the short sides. Stitch down.
- Thread a 6-inch-long, 1/8-inch-wide piece of elastic through the full hem on each side of the mask and knot it, and this is one of your two ear loops. In case you do not have the elastic, you can use hair ties or rubber bands as an alternative material. In case you only have string or fabric, you can make the relationship longer and tie the mask behind your head. Pull-on the ear loops, so the knots are tucked inside the hem.
- At this point, you have to collect the sides of the mask on the elastic and adjust it so that the cover to your face.
- Now, stitch the elastic (or fabric) in place on the corner of the mask to keep it from slipping -

- and voila! You'veYou've seen a cover in six steps.

How effective are they?

The health department has determined that homemade fabric masks are not to be considered as valid and adequate personal protective equipment. (PPE) "However, homemade masks can be considered to all intents and purposes, an effective complementary tool to other various methods such as hand washing, social distancing, and other measures aimed at preventing respiratory infections."

"I think it's mostly that people might not become complacent, that they have a homemade mask on.

Fleece said: "Depending on what material they are made of, they can approach the effectiveness of disposable surgical masks."

"But in case you are not using the right material and practising excellent hygiene. "These efforts do nothing but have the negative potential to worsen the situation, providing a false sense of protection in people."

In addition to inappropriate filtering of particles and germs, some masks can also pose additional risks, mostly if we're reusing them. A critical 2015 study published in the medical journal "BMJ OPEN" highlights the risk deriving from the improper use of fabric masks, highlighting how some parameters such as:

"the presence and retention of humidity, inadequate reuse, and imperfect alteration can Significantly affect the increased risk of infection."

So, to use them safely, it is appropriate to use them with logic, awareness, and responsibility, to try to create a sort of barrier between the sick and the healthy.

Is there a way to make better masks?

An influential 2013 study performed by the University of Cambridge states that " the type of material used for homemade masks can have an influential impact on their effectiveness." Also, according to the data analyzed by the same study, some materials are to be considered valid options for the production of a mask, thanks to their ability to help block and filter some virus particles from infected people. Among these articles we need: cotton blend shirts and antimicrobial pillowcases, kitchen tea towels and vacuum cleaner bags

Are homemade masks effective for healthcare workers?

Levine said in a press conference that: "Compared to N95 respirators, or surgical masks, fabric masks are less effective, but they may be better than nothing.

He also acknowledges their inadequacy if provided to healthcare professionals." Naturally, he points out that the fabric masks are not right to use and give to the medical staff employed in the treatment of patients with COVID-19.

According to the words of Ashish K. Jha, the top representative of the Harvard Global Health Institute, the medical community accepted with irony and mockery the recommendation on the use of the bandana by the CDO. Always what Jha said:

"In the presence of a potentially lethal and infected droplet, no evidence has been found that makes the bandana a valid method to protect the doctors and that therefore, in general, it is necessary to protect them with adequate medical protection."

Concerning homemade masks, the CDC also expressed its opinion, not considering them as proper personal protective equipment, as the effectiveness is unknown and is not well established by any evidence. If this decency continues, this will have an impact on healthcare workers, who would thus have few alternatives.

In that case, other options would be considered, which at that point would become necessary.

According to chief medical information offer at Temple University Hospital, David Fleece, "if nothing changes, and there are still evident difficulties in finding the masks, in a short time we will and ourselves without supplies equipment for protection from virologic infections, from which to draw."

According to Fleece, therefore, if nothing should change on the offer side, that of the hand-sewn mask, which is now considered only as an alternative, over time, it could take on greater prominence and be more used.

Can hospitals accept donated masks?

Following the worsening health situation, some hospitals have decided to accept donations of homemade cloth masks.

Still, however, these are sporadic cases, so, before producing a batch of masks to be donated to hospitals, it is advisable to inquire through the local medical facility, if they eventually accept donations.

A striking example was when the Philadelphia Emergency Management Office placed an announcement highlighting the call for help to address the urgent need for surgical masks, especially medical that are not made at home.

Penn Medicine and Jefferson Health are also not accepting homemade mask donations, excluding at least provisionally the acceptance of voluntary contributions of masks sewn at home.

Meanwhile, some organizations, among which the names of Masks for Heroes, and Masks for Docs in Indiana, are proceeding to directly connect the producers and suppliers of masks, with the operators and health institutions that request and accept donations, such as Sew Face Masks Philadelphia.

Whether you are a supplier or a requester, this section is dedicated to those interested in creating or receiving masks, who can check the database to forms to provide or receive covers via the websites of these groups. Preferential in delivering or receiving facial masks.

Always Fleece says that one of the structures in the

Philadelphia area, belonging to the health system of Temple University, accepting any donations of do-it-yourself masks. Although evaluation plans have not yet been put in place as to whether and how these donations will be used Currently, Temple Health is corned among the health bodies registered with Mask for Heroes, to facilitate the mask donation procedures that the latter makes available to health bodies. Another institution who said he agreed on future donations of homemade masks, if necessary, was the Philadelphia Children's Hospital, which welcomes new announcing for interested persons to make donations mentioned above, sending them into the structure (3401 Civic Center Boulevard) or let them directly in the main lobby of the hospital itself.

Also, in Fleece's opinion, there is a good chance that homemade masks should also be used, in case the supply of protective devices should continue on this path.

Should I wash my mask?

According to Nate Wardle, the press secretary of the Pennsylvania Department of Health, using detergent and hot water is the most effective method for proper washing of homemade masks. While to dry them, it would be necessary to use techniques that provide drying at high temperatures, to kill all germs and bacteria.

What type of ties do you want?

There are currently several ways to tie a mask to the face, but three main ways will be explained, planned, and illustrated here.

The ties that go around your ears. These are loose ties that you tie together behind your ears each time you put the mask on. This is simplest to make and requires the least work upfront, but you'll need to tie the cover each time you wear it. You can merely slip it on.

Ear-loops. Elastic may be better than fabric for this style since you'll need the ties to be short and tight enough to stay securely wrapped around your ears, but not so quick and close that they pop off.

The ties that go around the back of the head. You'll want the relationship to be long enough to go around the end of the head horizontally, but short enough that the t won't be too loose.

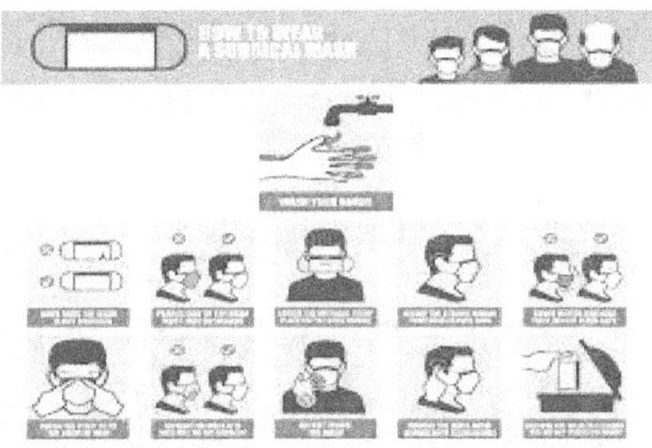

CHAPTER 6: BUILDING AN EFFECTIVE FACE MASK

First Step: Cut two pieces of fabric You want two rectangles, 12 inches wide, and six inches tall Our template is already the right size, so you can just cut out our model, then cut the fabric to t.

Second Step: Sew the fabric rectangles together

Sew the pieces together as tightly as possible. Go along all four sides, about 1/4" to 1/2" from the edge.

Using the template: Place the model on top of the two pieces of fabric and sew all three layers together along the dotted line.

Third Step: Cut fabric or elastic ties. Cut the links to the right size. If you're using fabric ties, you may want to cut wide strips that you can then fold in to hem. That would help keep them from fraying and falling apart when washed.

Fourth Step: Sew the fabric ties to the mask Tightly sew the ends of the fabric ties to the corners of the cover. On the template, sew the links to the marked boxes. For ear loops, create one loop on the left and another on the right, attaching one end at the top of the mask and one end at the bottom.

The forties that go around the back of your head sew each of the four ties to different corners, long enough so that you can tie them behind your head when you put the mask on.

The forties that connect behind your ears, simply sew each of the four ties to different corners.

Fifth Step: Sew around the entire edge again.

Do another pass around the entire outer edge of the mask, ensuring a tight seal between the two pieces of fabric and also securing the ties even further. On the template, sew along the second dotted line.

That's it! Remove the template, if you' you're using it, and your mask is ready to go.

Three ways to upgrade the mask

We have shown you how to make a simple

mask, using the advice suggested by the Pennsylvania Department of Health. But, in case, if you have a little more skill and patience, here you can end three exclusive ways with which you can update the mask:

First, let's start by dipping the mask inside-out instead of leaving the raw edges. In this way, having the frayed edges inside could help keep the cover together and not degrade while being washed. It also looks more beautiful. To do this, the best thing to do will be to sew the ties on one layer, then superimpose the second layer on top of it. At this point, you need to stitch the two layers of fabric together, leaving one or two inches of space instead of completing a complete rectangle. Now, ip the mask inside-out through that rectangle, then sew around the outer edge again.

Fold horizontal pleats. This allows the mask to better the curvature of your face, similar to how surgical masks work. The New York Times has a guide of its own, to make a mask with pleats and that you IP inside-out.

Use the third layer. Some expert seized the opportunity and recommended having two layers of material, but some projects even use a third disposable layer to help better filter the air. Those can include elements that can show them, such as Swiffer disposable dusting pads, coffee filters, paper towels, or something similar. Suzanne Willard, the dean of global health at the Rutgers School of Nursing, says she also uses masks at home using disposable liners.

What to do when you don't have sewing materials:

Remember, homemade masks aren't perfect. So, don't worry about doing everything right as we suggest that the point is to create a crucial mask that covers the nose and mouth, adhering well to the face.

As an alternative method to sewing, you can in case use materials such as safety pins or some clips, to keep the fabric and the bands together. Or staple everything together if necessary.

Don't have the possibility to connect fabric and ties? Don't worry, CDC has non-stitching options in the mask and uses something else. A scarf or bandana can be used if you can make or buy a cover, some tricks to keep in mind about your homemade mask:

First of all, you need to disinfect the mask between every use. The most effective way is to wash it with the rest of the laundry, in hot water and with soap or detergent, then pass it through the dryer and dry in warmer temperatures.

When you are a frequent user, depending on your needs or the type of work and social context you belong to, you may need to create more than one mask, depending on how often you go out.

Take the mask off carefully. Wash your hands before taking the cover off and assume the virus is being collected on the front of the hood. Remember never to touch the front part directly, because the method to remove it properly is with the ties. Remember not to touch your face. Also, wash your hands often even after unmasking.

Masks don't guarantee perfect protection. The use of a cover does not give you the freedom to think of being immune and able to get in touch with others without the risk or otherwise take irresponsible and risky behaviour.

The best behaviour to adapt and continue to stay at home as much as possible and keep the right social distance from others when you leave home.

Is there the best material for a reusable face mask?

However, the best fabric for homemade masks par excellence is a tightly woven, made of 100% cotton fabric. Some interesting ideas for making cotton products is to draw on materials such as sheets, curtains, and woven shirts, considered valid options if they are made entirely of cotton. If you intend to donate the masks, it is highly discouraged the use of knit fabrics (e.g., jersey T-shirts) for the real reason that by stretching, they create holes, which the virus could easily pass. To kill germs and pre-shrink the material, prewash the fabrics with hot water so that it does not change shape after users wash it themselves.

The things you need on top of a sewing machine and fabric are a non-woven interface for reusable masks, intending to block the particles appropriately, then elastic bands or ties to secure it correctly on the face and a piece of metal (like a paperclip) to t it comfortably around the nose without the risk of it slipping away from it. In case you cannot and an interface, you can modify an existing non-woven product, such as HVAC filters or coffee filters, but keep in mind that if you use one of these occasional products, it is better not to use the masks produced as donations if they are not washable. HEPA vacuum bags are also non-woven with functional alteration capabilities; just make them don't contain bar-glass

The beautiful thing about being able to reuse and reinvent products that you already have at home is that you don't have to spend more money to buy them. If you have clothes at home that you no longer use or bed linen, you can very well use them instead of having to buy new fabric. On top of that. All 860 stores offer materials in their classrooms with sewing machines, which, according to the company company's requests, will follow the appropriate recommendations on social distancing. In case you already own a sewing machine, if you prefer not to enter the shop for safety, you can also contact the shop directly, and have the supplies delivered directly outside your car, for a comfortable and safe collection on the sidewalk.

There's also been a buzz around shop towels (usually used by auto mechanics) after a group of seamstresses said they could filter particles better than other at-home face mask materials. As medical laboratories have not yet tested them, they are not however recommended by the CDC, at this point, you can stick with a tightly woven cotton fabric, along with two layers of a non-woven interface. One of the most popular products by women to make a reusable mask is the Hepa vacuum bags.

Young woman with fabric samples for curtains at the table. Multiple colour fabric texture samples selection fabrics for interior decoration. Furniture upholstery

CHAPTER 7: WILL HOSPITALS ACCEPT HOMEMADE MASKS?

Currently, homemade masks are not approved by hospitals, which, with exceptions, will not accept donations of this kind. Check and inquire with the local hospitals in your area if they have provisions to use homemade masks and, if so, what are their procedures they adopt to dispose of them. We must, therefore, consider the rapid evolution of the situation, and the various updates that hospital bodies use to deal with the health emergency.

In unusual cases, if they need it, healthcare professionals are also making requests on social media. There are various portals, which publish these IPR requests from healthcare professionals within social communication channels, such as Instagram pages and groups, Facebook. One of these portals, or Masks for Heroes, which uses an Instagram page to promote IPR requests, and to achieve this goal. To deal with the emergency, some hospitals are said to have given consent to their healthcare workers to send these requests, but with the demand for full anonymity of their identities. There is an institution, The U.C.

Does it make sense to wear a homemade mouthguard?

Medical protective equipment is urgently needed in nursing and is, unfortunately, also in short supply here. That'sThat's why you see more and more self-made protective masks on the streets and in shops - but do they make any sense, and do they protect the wearer from possible infection? In the following, we explain how the homemade protective masks work and what you should pay attention to.

Does a condent breathing mask protect against infection?

A self-made mouthguard cannot be compared to an FFP2 mask, which protects against aerosols and droplets. A self-made breathing mask does not protect the wearer from infection. However, wearing a makeshift oral and nasal mask can help curb the spread of the coronavirus. Although the cover does not protect the wearer, it serves as a blockage. This means that the wearer of a respirator mask can protect others from infection because pathogens are at least partially retained by the barrier. This is particularly useful if the required distance of two meters cannot be maintained, for example, when shopping.

Necessary: Even if you wear a mask, you should keep your distance, and the hygiene measures (washing and disinfecting hands regularly) take into account.

DIY mouthguard: what should you pay attention to?

It is essential that the mask consists of tightly woven cotton fabric (several layers) and is washed regularly at a minimum of 60 °. It should be cleaned after each wear - so it makes sense to make several masks at once. Please only wear the covers for a short time (e.g., for the time of shopping) and never all day, otherwise incredible viruses can accumulate here. The respirator mask is even safer with an insert that can be replaced (e.g., kitchen paper or hygienic

Fleece (e.g., high alteration vacuum cleaner bag, sponge cloth with clean coating, etc.) see also sewing instructions. Both patterns are designed so that an insert is no problem can be added and exchanged.

Models of protective coatings for the face and face masks:

Currently, there are three main types of protective coatings for the face: fabric, surgical and N95 respirators. Facial fabric coverings are the only coatings that are recommended to wear for the public. While the other models mainly concern health workers.

Fabric face coverings are generally, face coverings, made with household items or made at home with low-cost common materials, which are often already present in our homes.

A cloth face-covering is a facial protective cover to protect and prevent the virus from spreading by moving from those who do not wear it to other healthy people or without symptoms.

Surgical Masks are facial protective covers, typically used in the health sector.

They are used to prevent the risk of infection from infected droplets in the air and ensure protection from all germs except the small particles may carry coronavirus, which, they manage to go beyond them anyway.

N95 Respirator Masks, also called medical respirator masks, are perfectly tight setting respiratory masks for the face, reserved strictly for health professionals who work in close contact with patients with respiratory infectious diseases and protect them from airborne and fluid hazards. They significantly reduce exposure to particles, including small particle aerosols and large droplets. N95 masks manage to filter at least 95% of the particles suspended in the air.

CHAPTER 8: GUIDELINES FOR WEARING A FACE-COVERING

Improper use of face shields can lead to breathing and the emission of harmful air particles through the mouth and nose. In this way, there is an increase in contracting and spreading the virus to other people.

Your face covering should: tight snugly but comfortably against the side of your face be secured with ties, or ear loops include multiple layers of fabric allow for breathing without restriction be laundered and machine dried without damaging or changing the shape.

Putting on your face covering

Step 1 – Wash your hands with soap and water or an alcohol-based hand sanitizer.

Step 2 – Inspect your face covering for holes or tears.

Step 3 – Place covering over your mouth, like so:

With Ear Loops: Hold by ear loops and place a circle around each ear with Ties:

Bring to your nose, place ties over the crown of your head, and tie.

Step 4 – Pull the covering over the bridge of your nose, mouth.

Making your cloth face mask

You can make your cloth face mask with everyday items around the house and a sewing machine.

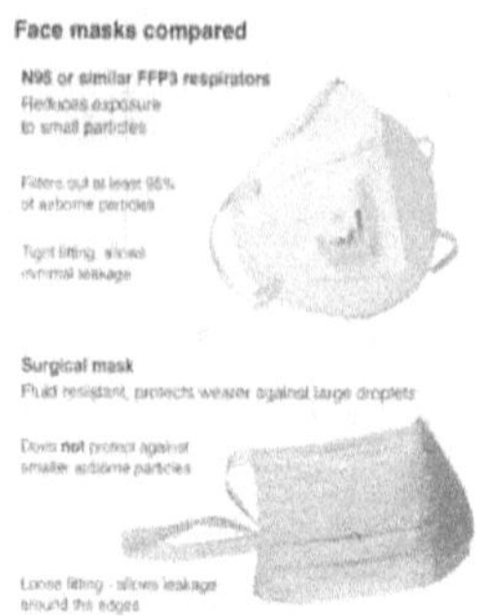

What you'll need:

Two 10" x 6" rectangles of cotton fabric from a t-shirt, scarf, or

Towel Two 6" pieces of elastic or rubber bands, string, cloth strips, or hair ties

Needle and thread, or bobby pin

Scissors

Sewing machine

Steps

1. Stack the two pieces of fabric together and sew them into a single piece of cloth.
2. Fold the long sides ¼ inch and hem.
3. Fold the double layer of material over ½ inch along the short sides and stitch down.
4. To make ear loops, run a six-inch length of elastic through the opening of the broader hem

on each side. Use a needle or bobby pin to thread through.

5. Tie the ends tightly.
6. Gently tug the elastic, so the knots are tucked inside the hem.
7. Stitch the elastic in place so, it doesn't slip.

Do I need a filter?

The purpose of a filter is to partially or entirely block the access and exit of potentially infected particles contained in the air coming from and directed towards our respiratory tract. It is possible to increase the altering capacity of a face mask homemade, adding to it an additional layer of propylene, acting as a filter. Propylene is a ubiquitous material in our homes, which can be found in ordinary shopping bags.

The need to add the filter between layers of cotton or other fabric can be seen as an essential precaution to ensure that the beers do not enter our lungs.

Why are face masks necessary?

Facemasks help limit the spread of germs and bacteria. When someone talks, coughs or sneezes, they can release small particles of saliva into the air, that can infect others. An effective face mask can reduce the number of germs released by the wearer, and it can serve to protect others from the risk of being infected when they come into close contact with infected individuals.

CHAPTER 9: HOW LONG DOES A DISPOSABLE MASK LAST?

The type of disposable mask, that built with a strap over the head. This model guarantees very little protection from debris and particles from the atmosphere. These dust masks, as illustrated above in the gore, also take the name of nuisance dust masks and are used in operations such as blowing the leaves to protect themselves from domestic debris. Dust masks just don't offer an excellent face seal and protect well as nose hair, which is to say not that well. It is recommended to replace them when breathing becomes difficult, or after about 8 hours of use and in the presence of exploitation.

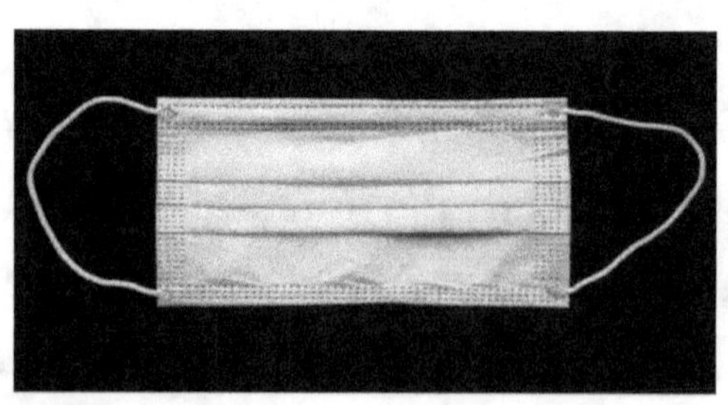

Replace them immediately and often whenever they start to get dirty, damaged, or make breathing difficult, which happens continuously in a construction site where the masks often get dirty the moment you put them down. Molded creates disposable respirators with an exterior lightweight plastic mesh, which helps keep the right filter cloth from contact with dirty surfaces. These masks arrive from the Molded 2200 model that does not always have a breathing valve or the Molded 2300 version, which does possess the exhalation valve. The lid helps maintain the wearer somewhat more relaxed during long periods of working in the mask.

Being able to breathe through a disposable respirator can be very difficult if the filter material becomes clogged or dirty. This is another main reason for improving them. Also, to solve this problem, a practical solution has been devised simply by creating more overlapping surfaces and obtaining more excellent altering. Even the modelled airwave includes an accordion surface that prevents both from getting too dirty and by inserting alter material inside the front area, to guarantee a longer duration, where it takes longer before it is clogged again.

Dust masks and disposable respirators, if damaged and, with torn parts, will have to be changed, as they have a particular purpose to be completed and, if they have perforated sections, they will let in what they should instead alter.

What happens most often is one of the belt breaks. In some cases, it is solvable, while in others, it is to be thrown in the trash and replaced with a new mask.

Another thing to think about is germs. Don't talk about dust masks. Most people do not like to try this anyway. But even when your disposable respirator (or dust mask, also if you are still using one next short article) sounds good after a lot more than just a day, change it out anyway. Many disposable respirators have antimicrobial surfaces, but over the years that they could start to be considered home to germs. Change them out after 8-10 hours, and even if they're, they're not cluttered.

Only recently, the CDC decided to take a drastic stance on the COVID19 pandemic, announcing his concern about the evolution of events, and the fact that it is considered necessary for each person to start wearing face masks in public.

One person who was one of the prominent exponents to have approved the use of the mask immediately is Jeremy Howard, an illustrious researcher at the University of San Francisco. In addition to the profession of skilled and experienced researcher he holds at the University of San Francisco, he is recognized as the founder of fast.ai, a research institute dedicated to making deep learning more accessible. His idea was to have created the Masks4all.co portal, in which he uses and promotes the benefits of everyone in the use of face masks, including those made at home.

CHAPTER 10: HOMEMADE FACE MASK

Surgical masks and respirators of the N95 type are considered to be medical devices, and reserved purely for healthcare and hospital use, for all those who respond in the first person to the need to come into contact with coronavirus patients.

For other people, it is the use of non-medical masks, so even those made at home are more than good.

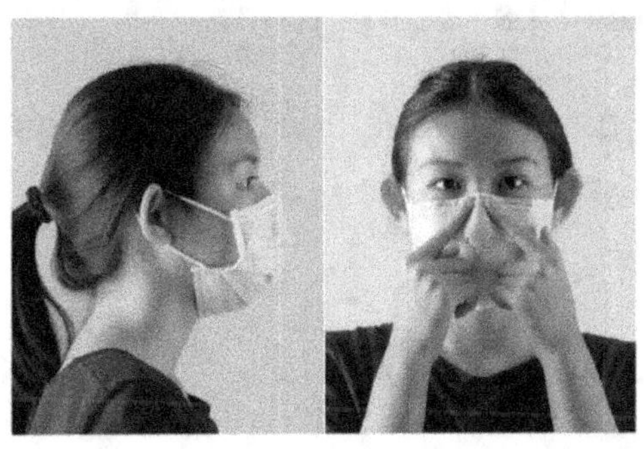

What is really important to know:

Homemade masks are suitable for providing generic protection for yourself, your family, and the people around you, in situations where it is difficult to maintain the task of social distancing, for example, on public transport, in grocery stores, etc.

Given for sure the presence of people with coronavirus, but asymptomatic or who before developing the mild symptoms, still manage to spread the viral infection to others.

For this reason, it should be a good habit that everyone, without exception, uses a face mask.

The homemade masks do not guarantee full safety for the wearer. Still, at least they are better than nothing and manage to protect and prevent only relatively, the risk of spreading and contagion of viral particles.

Everyone must follow the suggestions for using the mask correctly to take advantage of it and safety. These valuable tips recommend:

To improve their hygiene and adopt the good habit of washing their hands before wearing and removing the mask.

Another recommendation to keep in mind is never to

touch or adjust the mask without having adequately cleaned and disinfected your hands.

Don't reusing a cover once you have put it on.

Once used, keep them safe until they can be cleaned with warm, soapy water.

Note: Important thing to know is that non-medical masks alone will not eliminate the risk of spreading COVID-19. Everyone must be aware that they must rigorously adopt adequate hygiene and public health measures so that respectful and responsible behaviour must be maintained, and more outstanding care must be taken for personal hygiene with frequent washing and physical spacing measures to increase the level of safety.

Using Homemade Face Masks Safely

Homemade masks have limitations of use restricted to secure contexts where the risk of contagion is not excessive and to ensure better protection, and they must be safe. For example, those who work in hospitals where the risk of infection is higher will not use DIY masks. You, but the surgical model. Non-medical face masks or facings must be placed on:

Children under the age of two anyone who has

trouble breathing

Anyone who is incapacitated, unconscious, or otherwise unable to remove the mask without appropriate precautions and assistance.

When you choose to use a homemade face mask:

Keep attention to wash your hands immediately before wearing it on and quickly after removing it, and therefore practice good and adequate hand hygiene while wearing it.

Ensure the mask is snug against your face and that it has no damaged parts, such as holes or torn fabrics.

Never share your face mask with other people, because you cannot know if the other person is infected. Furthermore, it is not necessary to wear it and remove it repeatedly during a single use because it increases the risk of accumulation of bacteria and germs onThe masks can be easily contaminated, when they come into contact with the external environment, or when touched by your hands. When wearing a mask,

CHAPTER 11: TAKE THE FOLLOWING PRECAUTIONS TO PROTECT YOURSELF

When using a mask, you should avoid touching it unless necessary. The moment the cloth mask becomes damp or gets dirty, replace it immediately with a new one, For washing homemade fabric masks, it is recommended to wash them in the washing machine, also together with other objects. Just use washes with hot wash cycles, placing them in a mesh bag to avoid asking during washing at high temperatures, As for the non-medical facial masks that cannot be washed. It is required to replace and dispose of them as soon as they become damp, stained, or crumpled.

How to properly dispose of masks in a lined garbage can:

Don't leave used face masks in shopping carts, on the ground, etc.

They are making Homemade Face Masks Use clean and stretchy 100 per cent cotton t-shirts or pillowcases. Some materials work better than others.

Make sure that the facial mask is perfectly adherent to the face by completely covering the nose and mouth, so as not to allow the passage of infected droplets.

The mask should be comfortable; otherwise, you won't want to wear it consistently.

CHAPTER 12: MAKING DIFFERENT FACE MASKS WITH EXPLANATIONS AND ILLUSTRATIONS

Origami Cotton Fabric Mask

Tutorial

1.   First of all, start to cut out two 10-by-6-inch rectangles of cotton fabric.

Then, use tightly woven cotton, such as quilting fabric or cotton sheets. T-shirt fabric will work in a pinch. Stack the two boxes; you will sew the mask as if it was a single piece of cloth.

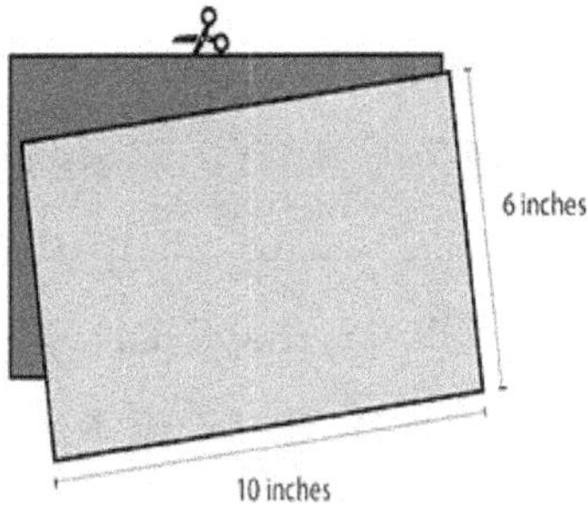

A close up of the two rectangular pieces of cloth needed to make a cloth face covering is shown. These pieces of fabric have been cut using a pair of scissors, each part of cloth measures ten inches in width and six inches in length.

2. Fold over the long sides ¼ inch and hem. Then fold the double layer of fabric over ½ inch along the short sides and stitch down.

.   Fold over the long sides ¼ inch and hem. Then fold the double layer of fabric over ½ inch along the short sides and stitch down.

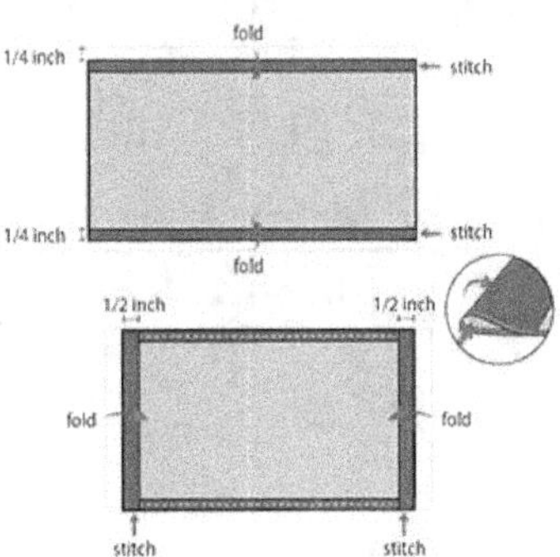

The top diagram shows the two rectangle cloth pieces stacked on top of each other, aligning on all sides. The rectangle, lying at, is positioned so that the two ten-inch sides are the top and the bottom of the box, while the two six-inch sides are the left and right side of the rectangle. The top diagram shows the two long edges of the cloth rectangle are folded over and stitched into place to

create a one-fourth inch hem along the entire width of the top and bottom of the square. The bottom diagram shows the two short edges of the cloth rectangle are folded over and stitched into place to create a one-half inch hem along the entire length of the right and left sides of the face covering.

3.   Run a 6-inch length of 1/8-inch wide elastic through the full hem on each side of the mask. These will be the ear loops. Use a large needle or a bobby pin to thread it through. Tie the ends tight.

Don'tDon't have elastic? Use hair ties or flexible headbands. If you only have a string, you can make the relationship longer and tie the mask behind your head.

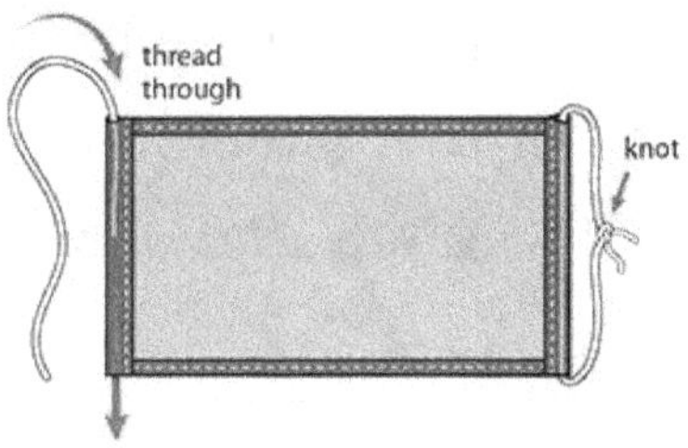

Two six-inch pieces of elastic or string are threaded through the open one-half inch hems created on the left and right side of the rectangle. Then, the two ends of the flexible or rope are tied together into a knot.

4. Gently pull on the elastic so that the knots are tucked inside the hem. Gather the sides of the mask on the flexible and adjust, so the cover it'sits your face.

Then securely stitch the elastic in place to keep it from slipping.

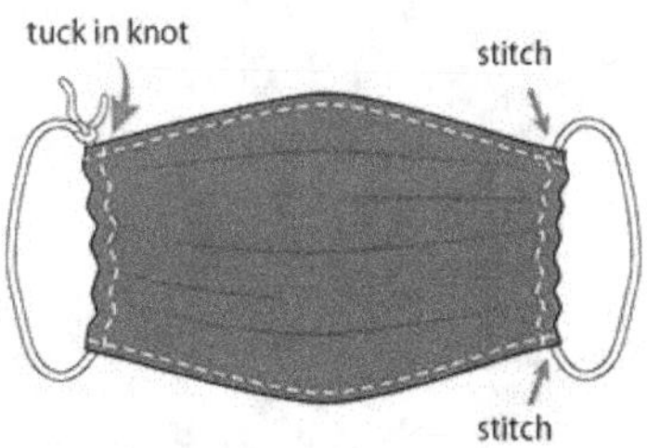

The diagram displays a completed face covering, in which the knots of the elastic strings are tucked inside the left and right hems of the mask and are no longer visible. The cloth is slightly gathered on its left and right sides, and additional stitching is added to the four corners of the gathered cloth rectangle, at the points where the cloth and the elastic or string overlap in these corners.

Creative Cloth Mask

Materials

- T-shirt Scissors
- Tutorial

A front view of a T-shirt is shown. A straight, horizontal line is cut across the entire width of the T-shirt, parallel to the T-shirt'sT-shirt's waistline. Using scissors, the cut is made approximately seven to eight inches above the waistline, the front and back layer of the T-shirt is cut simultaneously.

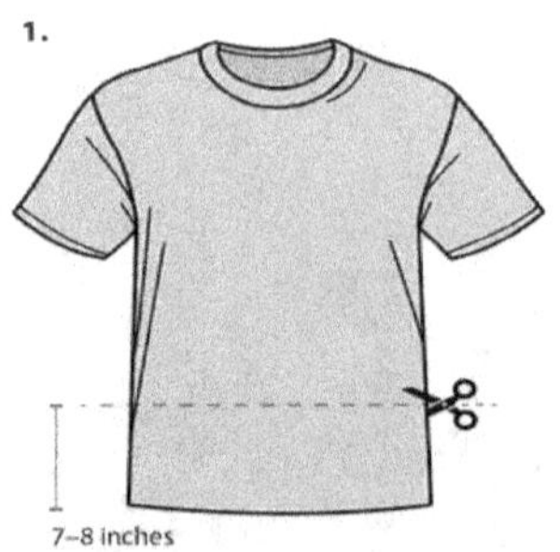

The rectangle piece of cloth that has been cut from the bottom portion of the T-shirt is shown, lying at. The rectangle is positioned so that the cut that was just made across the entire width of the shirt is the top side of the box, while the original waistline of the

T-shirt is the bottom side of the rectangle. From the top right-hand corner of the square, the scissors are moved down an approximately one-half inch, along the right, hemmed side of the box. From this point, a six to seven-inch, a horizontal cut is made through both the front and backside of the cloth, parallel to the top of the rectangle. The scissors then turn ninety-degrees to cut downward, a vertical line that is parallel to the left side of the box; this cut continues downward until it reaches approximately one-half inch above the bottom of the rectangle. The scissors then turn ninety degrees again to create another six to seven-inch, horizontal cut that runs parallel to the bottom of the box, back towards the right hemmed side of the shirt and cuts through the power hemmed side of the rectangle. This newly cut out piece of cloth is laid to the side. To cut the tie strings, the two remaining slivers of the right side of the rectangle are cut vertically along the hem.

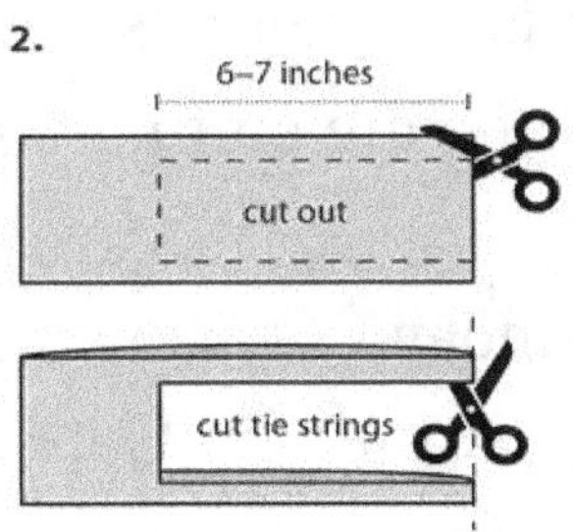

The piece of cloth is unfolded and worn by an individual. The middle of the cloth piece is positioned to cover the nose and mouth area; the four thin slices of cloth act as tie strings to hold the cloth face-covering in place. The ropes around the neck, then over the top of the head, are tied into knots.

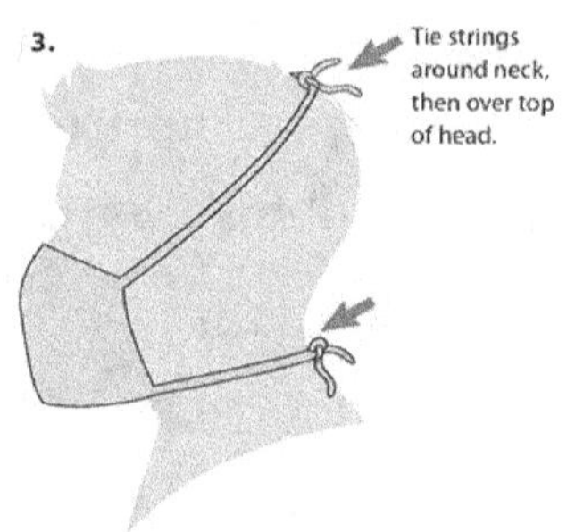

Bandana Protective Mask

Materials

- Bandana (or square cotton cloth approximately 20" x20")
- Rubber bands (or hair ties)
- Scissors (if you are cutting your fabric)
- Tutorial
  A single bandana is shown lying at, with the curved edge at the top. Cut banana in half with a horizontal line.

Fold bandana in half.

The square bandana is shown lying at. The bandana is then folded in half, bringing the top edge of the bandana to meet the bottom edge of the bandana.

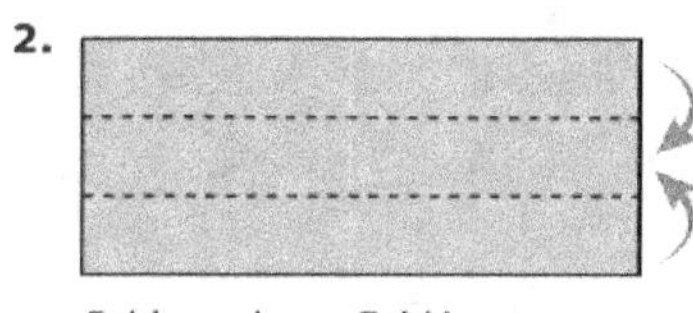

Fold top down. Fold bottom up.

The top half of the bandana, with the curved edg

e at the top, is placed in the centre of the folded bandana. Then, fold filter in the centre of the folded bandana. Fold top down. Fold the bottom up to cover the screen entirely.

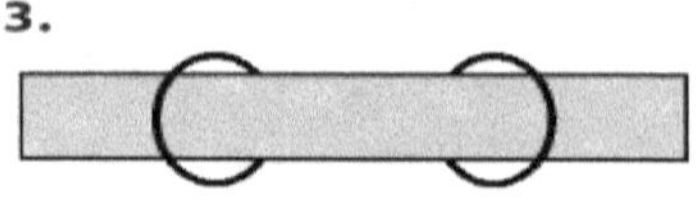

Place rubber bands or hair ties
about 6 inches apart.

Insert the folded bandana, with the filter inside, through the centre of two rubber bands or hair ties. Place rubber bands or hair ties about 6 inches apart.

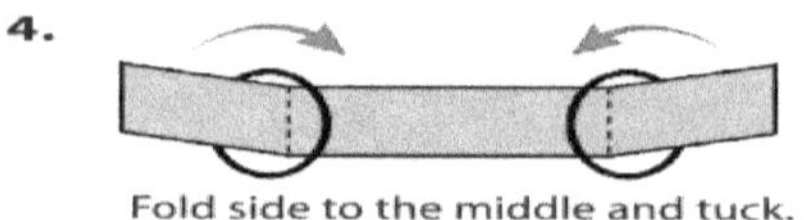

Fold side to the middle and tuck.

Take the left side and the right side of the bandana and fold each party to the middle and tuck the sides into each other.

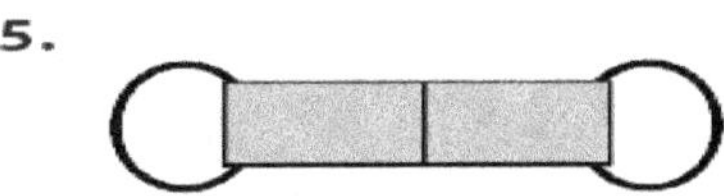

The bandana should now be a continuous, cloth loop since the left and right sides have been tucked into each other.

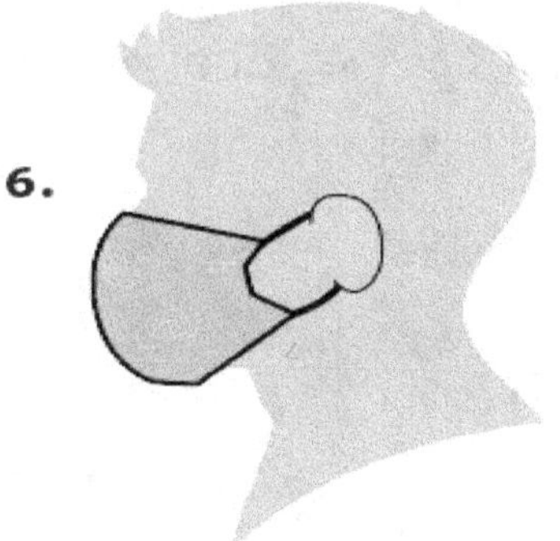

CONCLUSION

This book is all about the type of generally made mask, and use is likely to decrease viral exposure and infection risk on a population level, despite poor and imperfect adherence, personal respirators providing most protection. Masks worn by patients may not offer as high a degree of protection against aerosol transmission.